The True

Diamond Within

We have the power to heal others and oneself.

Vol 5

Extract from the original book,

'A Glimpse in a Transient Zone'

Jo Eaton.

Copyright.

Disclaimer.

The author of this book does not dispense medical advice or prescribe the use of any technique as a form of treatment for physical or medical problems without the advice of a physician, either directly or indirectly. The intent of the author is only to offer information of a general nature to help you in your quest for emotional and spiritual well-being. In the event you use any of the information in this book for yourself, which Is your constitutional right, the author and the publisher assume no responsibility for your actions.

In order to protect identity, I have changed the names of some of the characters within many of the stories.

Contents

Chapter 1

Healing Originated from

Caring for Others

From an early age, I know I have had a feeling of having to look after everyone. I remember at the age of three years; I began to comfort my Mum because she was upset. I knew I was role reversing even at that age. I felt in total control with the task of looking after my Mum. As time passed, I continued with this attitude, helping strangers who were in need, even organising days out for six children. For example, visiting the zoo or a day to the seaside, when at the time I was only ten years old. I was aware that the children never went on holiday and so I took the responsibility of organising transport, food and finance for the whole days out, even though some of the children were much older than I. Their parents said they were confident in my ability to look after the group and yet I am not sure why I felt I needed to take on this responsibility, but this caring theme in my life developed into trying to also heal my family if they were unwell.

Chapter 2

Hands on Healing;

Retaining emotional and spiritual distance when healing

I became aware that I was able to pass my hands over a sick person and then I felt a tingling sensation in the palms of my hand when I came across the problem area of the body. With a continuous passing over this area, wiping away any negative energy, then holding my hand over that problem part of the body, the tingling subsided. I would then 'hear' instruction as to how often to carry on with the treatment, receiving information as to what self-action the person should take to assist with the natural healing. This information seemed to be coming from an intelligence, higher than myself. I now know this kind of information is called channelling. I was always in an altered state of consciousness when performing this healing and yet it happened so quickly and naturally, I just accepted this was normal and it never ceased to help my family. Here are just a few examples:

- With just my hands hovering over Mike's troublesome knee, he called out in pain as he said it felt like a knife blade was being withdrawn from his knee. Thankfully he has had no more problem with this joint.

- My son in Australia had taken a fall and injured his foot, walking with a notable limp and so I performed healing on his foot while he read a book. Later, he commented he felt a pain in his foot during the healing, even though I was not exerting any pressure to the limb, but he too thankfully had no more problem walking.

- Our daughter wanted a natural birth, without medication and so when she went into labour, I worked with her contractions, performing Reiki on her lower back. We were doing very well until complications set in, due to the size of my grandson, which made a caesarean birth necessary.

This natural method of healing was taking place with friends and family about twenty-five years before I had any Reiki training.

With more practise over the years, my confidence increased and I then progressed to try to help other people outside the family, while encouraging them to look at the wider picture within their life, since I believe that the body will become sick if a problem in another area of your life has not been resolved. The symptom must be viewed holistically and not in isolation.

Any discomfort in your life or body, is information that you are not aligned with your true self. However, it is not always possible to make the appropriate changes to life's situations, but I always ask for guidance and follow any instruction given. Although the suggestions I have received does not always make sense at the time, in retrospect, it was sound advice.

I am also aware of the importance of hands. Subconsciously, I have always noticed peoples' hands in great detail, almost as much as their faces. In fact, I am able to recognise most people's hands who I have met. Since I use my hands when performing healing with light, I know it is important to clean your hands afterwards, by shaking and removing the other persons energy.

It was at the beginning of my Mum's long battle with terminal cancer when I became aware of the awakening of my healing ability. I had several years to think about life, about our purpose while we are here on earth and also the fragility of our mortality. This soul searching led me to the inner depths of spirituality and to start experimenting with healing. As a child, I had always been sensitive to my surroundings and to the emotional needs of others and yet, during those years of nursing my Mum, someone to whom I was profoundly attached emotionally, escalated my spiritual development. By this time, I had two small children and so I made a spiritual healing connection with our boys whenever they were ill, restless, or even when I was rocking them to sleep. It was very natural and appeared to always have a positive outcome, and so this practise began to be second nature to us within our family. (This was well before I had trained as a Reiki practitioner).

Throughout this spiritual journey, I have realised that it is very important for us not to give our power away to anyone. Observing healers working, I am aware they keep a certain emotional and spiritual distance in order that they are able to do their job. To an extent, doctors in the medical profession, also work in a similar way. When I try to give healing, I too maintain this sublime barrier because by giving your power away, then you become weaker and so not able to help yourself or others. It is a fine balance to achieve this state. We must also be constantly alert to the 'energy suckers', i.e. people who are drawing your energy. Having said that, it is very important to give unconditional love in abundance, since I believe we are love and constantly loved, as spiritual beings.

Chapter 3

When Healing Others You
Are Healing Self

Our past and future lives converge in the present, in order that we are moving towards a healthier and more spiritually fulfilled life. I am sure I have been an artist in a past life because from an early age I was always confident with such techniques, without being taught. So, maybe I am now preparing my work for future lives. I am aware of a shift in my art work, from becoming spiritually aware within the forest environment, to now incorporating my artwork to create healing environments, while now even being drawn towards sound, to increase the sensual experience. It is interesting to contemplate, as I move towards healing myself, I am also trying to heal others and the planet too.

Derived from mystical knowledge, I believe the soul is made up of several vehicles. For example, the causal body is the highest form of mind, being sensitive and fused with spirit, preserver of karma, intuition, and creativity. Memory, intellect and power is on a lower level, with the astral channel being the source of emotions and desires, which in turn, effects the physical body. This sublime body circulates energy around the individual, that is easily identified by clairvoyants, regarding the health of the person. This is why the body becomes sick, if there is an unresolved emotional problem. It is the body's way of making us deal with our problems, in order that the person returns to full health.

As we are so connected to each other, I think it is important to stay centred and to tell others about our path as it unfolds, while being of service and in doing so, knowledge is shared. Being spiritually connected, I have often come out with statements, not knowing why I was telling other people, or acting in such a way, sometimes to complete strangers, with the statements often sounding odd to me and yet had been a very relevant message and exactly what that person had needed to hear at the time. One such occasion was when a work colleague, Jenny, was very upset due to the recent death of her Mother. Jenny would often come into my classroom during our break-time to chat about her loss.

A short time later, when I was at home, I was aware of Jenny's Mum telling me to send a card to my friend, enclosing a button and a message, signed by her Mum. I was bewildered about the latter part of the request, but I still followed the instructions. I was rather apprehensive to give Jenny this card and message because I did not want to distress her even further.

Once I handed over the envelope, Jenny read the message and collapsed in floods of tears at the sight of the button. This was not the response I wanted, adding to my friend's grief and yet Jenny assured me they were tears of great joy. She knew the message was from her Mum. She then went on to explain that her Mum was a G.P. and on her desk in her surgery, was a dish where she collected buttons. Jenny knew I was not privy to this personal bit of detail but the button made great sense to Jenny, validating her Mum's 'presence' and so was part of the healing process.

Chapter 4

Nature is a Great Healer

As I progress on my journey, I have become more interested in sound being a vehicle for healing. Within the forest, there is the sound of the variety of birdsong, all competing for a solo performance, the running, gurgling of water, trickling over stones in the stream, the rustling of leaves in the trees, to the rhythm of the gusts of wind, the humming of the bees, as they gather nectar from the flowers. I find the birdsong of early Springtime a most spiritual experience. There are so many sounds in nature, if we only take time out to listen. This sound is very powerful and makes my heart sing. Everything in nature sings and vibrates in harmony, natures music. I believe there is a connection to spirit and soul, with each natural sound in nature, triggering vibrations in the atmosphere, while in turn, having a profound effect on man. Music is a force, giving off certain vibrations, depending on the type of sound.

On my Masters course, I was able to explore the idea of energies in nature even further, incorporating Albert Einstein's 'Theory of Everything' within my work, his idea of E=MC2, showing that there was no such thing as solid matter, but all things were made up of pure light energy. I understood from my teaching, that various cultures acknowledge this universal energy, having different names such as the Asian Prana, in China it is referred to as Chi, or Ki in Japan, all of which I incorporated within my work, with the aim of communicating my ideas across various cultures.

This clusters of energy emanates in nature, through humans too and actually surrounds us by way of auras. When healing with Reiki, meditating or using various Eastern traditions, often the practitioner or Shaman work with those auras, some being various colours, encircling the form, which denote the health and wellbeing of the patient.

Chapter 5

The Power of Sound

In my daily life, I often play spiritual, mediative music constantly throughout my home, since I am aware of the powerful vibrations within the atmosphere, creating a tranquil, positive and healing environment. One where I am able to have short moments of meditation to help with my creative ideas and how best to promote them, while improving personal health and increasing my spiritual advancement.

Many musicians have studied the science of psychology of sound and so understand that every sound has some effect on man, even a negative effect on the nervous system, with the wrong type of music.

I am aware of groups of 'Sound Adventures' now, meeting regularly, who collectively play a variety of music and sounds from various cultures, in an attempt to send healing to each other and in turn, sending positive vibrations out into the universe. Those groups certainly understand the importance and power of sound within music, to assist with the advancement of us beings on the planet.

For a long time, I have known of the healing power of sound too. I am aware that harsh, grating and shrill sounds are very negative and stressful to the human form, resulting in illness and yet soothing, harmonious sounds are conducive to healing. Many cultures around the world have used sound in this way for hundreds of years. For example, the

North American Indians used repetitive chanting to help with healing the sick; African tribes used drumming; while Buddhist monks still use chanting when meditating today. In fact, Patanjali, the Indian sage who lived more than one thousand and seven hundred years ago, composed words of wisdom, a system of medicine called Ayurveda and Yoga sutra, advising the repetition of the sound 'Aum' as clearing the mind while alerting your creative energy. The sound 'Aaah', when repeated, alters your form into the sound of creation.

Our response to sound is so fundamental to us humans and so this is one sense I am interested in exploring even further to include within my artwork, because I realise the power of those vibrations to help heal us. Today, there are many people making music to make contact with our divine vibrating energy waves, in order to help further our spiritual development.

The freedom I experience when dancing is one of ecstasy, one of great joy when moving your body to the rhythm of music, almost like being in a trance, in a world of your own. It is like in meditative state when you are in complete unison with your soul and since I was a small child, I have always enjoyed this experience. Although there is a great variation in sound and music, I imagine the sounds where you are able to 'lose yourself' must be congruent to your own vibration. This activity must be good for the soul since it is like celebrating life itself. All cultures seem to recognise this, from ancient times and even to those tribes using a basic drum beat. I believe it is inherent in human behaviour to move to sound. You just need to watch small babies who naturally sway and move to music or rhythmic sound.

Chapter 6

Other Techniques to Heal
the Body

Over the years, I have found other techniques to help me, in a natural way, to help harmonise and heal the body. For example, if I am unable to sleep, after meditation, then by just massaging the left earlobe for one minute, then I find I gently drift off to sleep. If I awake later in the night, then I just repeat the process so I fall asleep naturally, a much better method rather than taking medication.

In order to quell my nerves before an exam, I find it helpful to avoid a group of colleagues, who maybe taking the same exam, because I pick up on their nervous energies, compounding my situation. By withdrawing from the group, going for a walk, meditating then walking straight into the examination room, I have been able to arrive in a calmer demeanour, centralising my energy.

In his book, 'Creation: Artistic and Spiritual', the Bulgarian philosopher Omraam Mikhael Aivanhov explains there are other hand exercises too, that help calm the nerves. For example, stroke the back of your left hand, barely touching it with the palm of the right hand or stroke the fingers of the left hand in turn, with the three fingers of the right hand. There are even more hand exercises for they are like antenna which receives and transmits various energies. This is why it is important to frequently wash them in spiritual water throughout the day. It is quite easy to pick up unwanted energies throughout our day.

There is also a voluntary exchange of energy, whether it be used as a signal of attraction or when friends are having a fun time together. There follows a wonderful high after being in the company of such people.

It is interesting how grief has an effect over our bodies. Only nine months ago, I had a persistent cough. No matter what medication I used, nothing seemed to have any affect. I then turned to meditation, when I realised my cough was due to being distressed at the loss of my brother, who had passed more than two years earlier, but due to the legalities of a contentious case, I had not had the time to grieve. With the realisation of four months of mourning was enough, I released the emotion and the very next day, my cough had disappeared.

This same universal energy may also be used as an healing force, as in Reiki. It is possible, when meditating, to use this golden healing light to help others or yourself with a particular illness, to increase your energy, while in turn, travel to the injured parts of the body to help deal with the problem. I have had a lot of success with this method and it is so easy to learn and available to each of us.

I find it important to release past hurts and painful events in your life and replace them with forgiveness and love for yourself. This act of kindness will help to release negative thoughts and behaviour from past issues while allowing love to fill your life and sending this message out to others. You are then in a better position to allow and attract the positive energy of the Source into your life, in order to realise your desires and true destiny.

I have found it useful to look back on my life to see what activities have given me the most joy and pleasure and so I have made a conscious decision to try to reintroduce and incorporate those interests into my life. For example, I love creating, dancing, artwork, making textiles, socialising, travelling, quality time with my family and writing. If I am doing what I love, then I am happiest living in positivity, rather than dwelling on negative activities of complaining, gossiping, being critical etc. Negative thoughts and behaviour will block positive energy arriving to you and so I try to look for the good in others, rather than dwelling on the unpleasant behaviour or the troubles in the world.

We are able to heal with love and light through touch, but it is most important to speak in truth.

I make sure I surround myself with healing sounds, calming incense, while mediating to return to a high vibration. I try to exercise each day, eat good food, have clean drinks, meditate and foster peaceful surroundings in my home. I have noticed when I become engrossed in a creative activity, this helps greatly to heal and settle my body too.

This energy field, created by healing sounds and activities, raising vibrations, as I have been mentioning, not only vibrates around your home, around your town, your environment, around your county, your whole country and around the world. It is as a stone dropping in a lake, with the ripples moving outwards. Our vibrations are like sound waves, rippling outwards. This is why it is so important for each of us to take note when we shout and behave in anger. This negative behaviour has repercussions for everyone in the vicinity. We must all take responsibility for our actions and make an attempt to live in love and positivity on a higher vibration, for the good of all.

I remember being given some sound advice from one of my Tutors at University many years ago, after my attempts to address a social problem in another part of the world, within my painting. He said I needed to improve my own private world, while in turn, this would improve the world at large. If everyone participated in this activity, then the whole world vibration would increase and wars would be a thing of the past.

In her book, 'You Can heal Your life', Louise Hay believes every illness is the result of the mental cause of fear and disharmony. So, if we change our way of thinking, replacing negative thought patterns with positive ones, then the body will heal itself. Using this method, Louise explains how she cured herself after being diagnosed with terminal cancer.

On numerous occasions I have followed the advice suggested by Louise, whereby the majority of new thoughts encourage us to be at peace, that we are safe and all is well etc. As a result, we then start loving and approving of ourselves, and our body responds by returning to good health.

Our bodies are designed to heal and regenerate itself, if given time, but obviously there are times when we need medicine to assist our recovery to full fitness. However, I believe we need to take a holistic approach when healing, taking into account our spiritual, mental and physical well-being for the best results, because all our various energy vibrations need to operate in unison. If one of them are out of sync, then we have a problem.

For thousands of years, the philosophy of the Eastern medicine of Ayurvedic has been practised, where the patients are treated holistically, rather than localised. This idea is that the disease affects the body on a deeper level, and so the conscious mind is also treated. Some patients have taken an active responsibility in motivating their own healing, having a deep desire to live and yet today, when I visit the doctors, I rarely feel that they have understood me. They seem to address the problem in isolation, rather than holistically, failing to truly understand the body which depends on looking at your emotional and spiritual wellbeing, food intake, lifestyle, whatever else maybe going on in your personal life etc. There are so many areas of our life that may be contributing to our body being out of kilter.

I know our doctors are doing their best, under the time constraints, but I pick up on their uncertainty and lack of confidence, so I return home feeling I have not been heard correctly and that I have a much better understanding of my body. I do hope in the future our medical profession takes heed of the Ayurvedic tradition.

I believe our cells are extremely complex, within themselves, having an intelligence, memory, energy and a spark of the universal Source, and yet they are also vibrating in harmony as part of the whole, namely our body. It is almost playing in unison, as a beautifully tuned orchestra.

When our actions are matched with our emotions, then this results in a powerful empowerment, allowing us to fulfil our ambitions and goals in life. I find when I am in this mode of equilibrium, then I do not think of negative actions, not even thinking to control others, not being aware of anything other than the task in hand. When I am working in this state of concentration, I know my partner finds it difficult to even attract my attention.

This state of consciousness is working on a different level to the five senses of hearing, seeing, smelling, tasting and touching. It is a state of developing into an invisible multisensory experience of perception. I believe this to be a right brain activity, where the depth of concentration is like that of when in meditation, where you seem to lose track of time.

All our great mentors have been multisensory mortals who have been aware and able to tap into this advanced dimension. When operating on this multisensory level, we are never alone, being in closer contact with our guides, who lead us to work in love, compassion and wisdom. As we develop, then our multisensory perception allows us, through intuition, to 'read' other people. For example, you may intuitively know if someone is telling you lies, or if someone is behaving very stern, you just know that person is really warm inside.

However, I have been in a different situation where I have seen above the personality of someone else, then raised my perception to that of communicating soul to soul, and so, on a physical level, it may appear as if I have been rather weak, when in actual fact, I have been operating from a position of strength.

If there is a time in your memory when you felt lonely, unloved or frightened, then visit that small child in you and send loving thoughts to help heal the past negative emotions.

Chapter 7

Dealing with Irrational Fears

Many of our difficulties in life are caused by irrational fears. For example, fear of not being good enough, fear of not having enough money to pay our bills, fear of not securing a good job, fear of not being accepted by our friends, fear of not having the right body image, fear of change etc. The list is endless and yet those fears often are irrational and reduce our vibrations, resulting in negative energy. It is important to try to recognise this habit of cultivating unfounded fears, replacing them with positive thoughts and in doing so, raising your energy levels to a healthy optimum.

If you replace those negative emotions of fear, criticism, hurts, expectations and replace them with love, then somehow, the obstructions seem to disappear and life runs more smoothly. It is a matter of changing your mind set. To give you a simple example, when driving to town and you need a parking space, just imagine it to be there, just awaiting your arrival, and there it is. Otherwise, if you expect to be driving around town, looking for the non-existent space, then, chances are, you will not find one.

It is not necessary to have to prove yourself, not necessary to be afraid of what you want or do not have, just have the confidence to 'fly on your own'. I know this is easier said than done, because of commitments and responsibilities in your life, but for your wellbeing, it is important to lighten the load and look after yourself, to be kind to yourself, to love yourself and to be accepting on who you are. There have been many times when I know I have been underachieving in all aspects of life. I have many skills and I have attained some level of success, but I still feel I have not reached my full potential. Somehow, we feel we have to put things on hold, or give something up, in order to become acceptable to others. But this is not the case. We just need to constantly remind ourselves that we have the love and acceptance inside of us and so we do not need it from 'outside'.

I have been caught in this never-ending trap of trying to please other people and no matter how hard I try, I feel I have not met their expectations, resulting in a feeling of inadequacy. I now recognise this behaviour was in an attempt to receive from others their acceptance, love and admiration. Why do we need it when we are whole ourselves? This was a big turning point for me, a great learning curve to realise we are enough, just as we are. We must stop looking outside for love and acceptance, because we are love, if only we realise this fact. Our needs cannot be achieved by other people, but we may share our love with others in our life. Usually those who stay in a relationship through difficult times, are the ones who really love you because those experiences are helping you both to heal. If they leave the relationship before the problems have been resolved, then those same difficulties will resurface in yet another relationship until, eventually the circle of lessons have been completed, so enabling yet another cycle to begin.

Sometimes we do not make it clear what we want from others, and so we then end up with accepting conditions we did not want, possibly out of fear of losing that person. However, relationships are a way of learning lessons and then we are able to let go and move on, remembering to love ourselves unconditionally.

Throughout our life, there are times when we think 'outside the box' realising we are not on our life's path. It is then an opportunity to re-group our thoughts and draw up new aims, in order to realise our destiny.

Looking back, I gave up on pushing forward and instead, took a back seat, in an attempt to free-fall and just be in the 'now', to have faith in the cosmic flow, allowing spiritual intervention to direct my path. By this time, I had the courage to express myself, without fear of others' opinions and to remind myself I am not responsible for their actions. Even today, I still hear myself repeating this statement, almost as a reassuring affirmation.

I know I regularly discuss and share what I have learned with others. In fact, this is the whole idea of writing this book. Sometimes I am still confused about past dramas, not always having the answers, but then I know I am still in the healing process, working towards unconditionally loving self. I try daily to be the best person I can be, in an attempt to grow spiritually and in the knowledge, it is a work in progress, with the very things we are looking for, are within us.

Most of the time I do feel at peace, joyful, leading a life through service, and yet I just need to work more on living a life in abundance and fulfilment, in order to realise my full potential. Having said that, I know I am whole and 'inside', I know I have all the love I need. I do not have to impress anyone for their acceptance because I am enough, just as I am. I do things to help others voluntarily, through the act of service, not because I want something in return. I already have all I need. I have learned to accept myself, to take care of myself and take time out to be kind to 'me'. It is important, when looking at others, for us to try and forgive any wrongdoings and to be kind, seeing beyond any negative actions, in the knowledge that in the depths of each of us, there is a loving soul.

Whenever you feel fearful, you have depleted your energy and you are acting in a negative way, but by releasing fear from your life, this allows you to operate on a more even keel, one to operate in positivity.

I remember a time when I was very young, being left with an uncaring relative while my Mum was busy working, then looking after her sick sister. I felt very lonely and unloved and so I have had to work to eradicate those feelings in my soul memory, releasing the negativity and replacing it with warm, loving energy and emotions to that small child within, in the knowledge all is well. We are all able to delete fears of our past, removing any negative energy and replacing it with a new energy, full of healing, positive vibrations.

Chapter 8

Reiki and Similar Distant Healings

In this lifetime, I have become extremely interested in healing myself and also sending distant healing, through Reiki and similar distant healings. I noticed about fifteen years ago, when I had an operation under general anaesthetic, I knew there was a humorous banter going on between three male medics, during my operation. Although I was under the anaesthetic, I also knew we must be aware of what is happening to our body, almost as if we are an outward observer.

Another time, I knew of a friend who was about to embark upon a quadruple bypass operation, following a recent heart attack. I offered to send healing during the operation. Later, as I meditated, I found myself also in the operating theatre, observing the procedure. As I started to work on my friend, sending healing energy, I heard the surgeon comment how hot he felt and he asked the nurse about the temperature of the room because he felt so hot. At the time, I thought this was a strange request, as he was performing such a serious and complex operation. Although, at the time, I have since thought the heat may have been the surgeon picking up on the healing energy within the room.

Three days later, I received a surprise phone call from my friend, who was dialling from his home. I could not understand why he was not still in hospital. It transpires

29

his recovery was miraculous, and so he was released from hospital after only three days, following the major surgery. The usual recovery time following such an operation being a minimum stay in hospital of seven days. I mentioned to my pal, the surgeon's confusing conversation I heard during the operation, when my friend then explained that during heart surgery, the operating theatre needs to be kept at a very low temperature. I did not know this at the time, but now this makes sense of what I heard during the healing session. How wonderful for my friend that his recovery was so speedy. I am always in awe at the lovely natural way we are able to help heal each other, through Reiki or other methods of transference of healing energy. It is so important for us each to learn this very natural and non-invasive method of healing.

As part of this healing process, we must try to control our ego, in order to attain inner peace and joy. To foster feelings of love, forgiveness, not only for yourself but towards others and practise kindness, while eliminating fear, anger, greed and violence. It is then through meditation, looking within and spiritual development, that leads us on our spiritual journey towards enlightenment.

When I try to pass on certain wisdoms to others, there is a mixed response. Most listen with interest, maybe out of politeness, while others are more cynical. On one occasion, someone actually changed their opinion, listening intently and readily accepting Reiki to relieve a few problems. It maybe our soul shines through our eyes, because at times we each have an immediate connection with complete strangers, a sort of recognition, a knowing. So, I suggest our spiritual knowledge also emanates through our eyes.

Although I have been trained in healing with Reiki, I was aware I was able to heal many years earlier. I then realised, with help from your guides, you become a vehicle for the transference of energy, where you do not need to know how the healing happens, but it is more about your intentions, almost like you are channelling a spiritual energy. I once read about a North American Shaman describing it as 'hollow bones'. Somehow, this vibration is communicated to the person receiving the healing, then their own energy system takes over.

On my return to the UK, from a holiday in Germany, visiting my brother and his wife, I sent about four lots of distant Reiki healing to my sister-in-law, to help with her depression and as pain relief too, unbeknown to her. Later that week, I phoned my brother for a progress report on his wife. He could not believe the vast improvement in her health and noted, one day, she just rose from the sofa, feeling fine and promptly went on a bike ride while continuing to make great progress. Only then did I tell my brother about the Reiki healing, but my sister-in-law said it was just coincidence. That is fine, just as long as there was a positive outcome.

I have had the pleasure of meeting the healer Seka Nikolic, who runs world healing sessions. She arranges a time when interested people around the world, join together to send healing to each other and to our planet. This activity is acting in alignment, across all countries, religions and cultures, where the participants are consciously and collectively trying to make contact on a spiritual level, amplifying their intentions of not only healing themselves but the whole of civilisation and our Universe. This can only lead to a positive outcome, making our world a safer, peaceful, loving place. Almost collectively lifting the world to its ideal.

After taking both healing Reiki Levels One and Two, I experienced a period of discomfort, maybe because my aura and energy had been disturbed. It took about three weeks before I started to feel settled and so I made the decision not to advance to Reiki Level Three because I did not want to experience further disturbance. As I was able to help heal and send healing anyway, I decided not to pursue further levels, unless I was so guided.

While studying for my Master's Degree, there was a hardworking Technician in the Print Room who was struggling with severe back pain, most probably due to the continuous physical work on the presses and screen beds. We often spent our lunchtimes together and one day, he began to discuss his dream car, as an ex-rally driver and how he had a photograph of it on his bedside table, since it was far out of reach in reality, due to raising a family on a tight budget.

Eventually, this shy Technician accepted my offer of giving healing Reiki during one lunchtime, to help alleviate his back problem. I remember that during the session, my hands became burning hot. As I left University, I advised him to drink a glass of water before driving home.

It was a few weeks later, when we next met, only to be greeted by a very excited Technician. He explained, after receiving the Reiki, he was very relaxed and yet on his way home, someone was speeding in their car and crashed into the back of my friend's car, completely destroying it and yet my pal was miraculously unharmed, probably due to him being in such a relaxed state. As a result of this accident, compensation was paid out through the insurance company and so the Technician was now the proud owner of his dream car, even to the exact specification and colour of the car in his precious bedside photo. What a wonderful outcome.

Distant Healing

For years, a dear friend had been suffering discomfort with his knees but was reluctant to have an operation. I then offered to send distant Reiki, since he lived in another country, for seven days, in the hope of improving his situation.

I have kept a daily account of each procedure, without relaying the details to my friend, other than healing was being sent at 7.00am each day, for one week.

Day1. As I meditated, I was aware of being surrounded by several healers and Masters too, so I had to observe the psychic operation which was taking place, where a blue gel was inserted on the periphery of my friend's kneecaps, then 'cured'. Also, both of the outside of the upper and lower leg bones was being treated at the same time. Those bones were extremely damaged and jagged. After about ten minutes, the bones were returned into place. I was then aware of seeing my friend lying in bed, while his partner was fast asleep on the other side of the bed. I told my friend all was going well and gave him a hug before leaving.

Day 2. This time, I was told I would now need to do the procedure and so was handed a grey metal nozzle which held the blue gel. I was nervous at being given such responsibility, but the guides were very close by to offer support. I had to build up on yesterday's layer, a guide 'cured' it but I found it difficult to insert the gel between the two rubbing bones.

Afterwards, telepathically, I indicated to my friend he has a problem with fear and so his whole body needed the golden light. Before we left, my pal was still aware of our presence and of the sensation of being surrounded by light and love.

Later that day, I found myself feeling very low, being depleted of energy. When I meditated, I was told I needed to protect myself while healing and clearing my energy by wiping my hands of any negativity afterwards.

Day 3. Today, my friend was fast asleep. I had to insert a third layer of gel before another guide smoothed off the jagged bones, then sucking out any debris, to enable me to apply the gel over the total bone ends, before re-connecting and lining up the legs and the patellae. The guides then took over the procedure to complete and tidy up.

By this time, my friend began to stir from his sleep and as I gave him a farewell hug, he was very touched to realise that someone cared enough to try to help him.

Day 4. I had woken today at 5.30am and so fell asleep again. I was awoken by what sounded like a loud whoosh or sneeze sound in my right ear. I looked at my clock and it was exactly 7.00am. I shot out of bed; a bit startled because I had not heard that noise before. The guides were waiting for me. Once again, I continued with the distant healing process but was now given a type of brush to smooth over each area, after applying the gel. Due to being tired, I forgot to 'cure' the gel on the first patella, but I need not have worried because help was at hand.

Following the healing, I understood that there was some swelling since my friend had been lifting heavy items, because he felt so much better. I made a mental note to send an e-mail to remind my friend that only light duties are the order of the day, for the time being.

Wide blue bands were wrapped around each knee to act as a support and then my friend was surrounded by the golden healing light again. With eyes still closed, my pal asked for a hug, so he would know I was present and was instantly moved again, explaining he was overjoyed. I once again told him to release all fear because nothing or no-one can really hurt him. All is well.

Later that day, I sent an e-mail to remind him not to lift heavy weights because it would hamper the healing process.

Day 5. Today, I was awake earlier than usual and so I commenced the healing at 6.50am, when my friend abroad was fast asleep, actually awakening during the final five minutes of the session. The procedure was the same as

Day 4. but this time I was given full control, even lining up the leg bones and the patellae.

On completion of the process, the guides applauded my efforts and I had also been aware of the sound of angels singing high above, throughout the procedure. I was taken aback with this response.

I then spoke to my friend to remind him to 'kill the fear' because there are many people who love and care for him. No one or nothing can really harm him and so he needs to believe this, in order to relieve his asthma, eczema and anxiety symptoms. I know he hides his feelings behind a façade, but I see through it as if a pane of glass. All is well.

Day6. I started the session at 7.00am prompt, when I noticed the patellae no longer needed any gel, just gentle brushing over the new layers on each bone joint. Then I was instructed to insert a small amount of gel at the top, bottom and sides of each leg bone, once they were lined up in the correct position. Once again, a blue wrap was applied to each knee, for additional support, cooling and to help reduce any swelling. Tomorrow, the final day, only the gel would be inserted either side of each bone, filling any gaps. Again, I could hear angels singing in the distance.

Finally, my friend was showered in healing golden light, while I was encouraged to talk to him for reassurance. As he was beginning to stir from his sleep, I whispered in his ear and told him to release fear. He then communicated telepathically saying this past week he had felt very happy and cared for. Once again, I reminded him about the many people who loved and cared for him. My friend then asked how many were in attendance to the healing sessions. When I replied about ten Masters and guides, he was very moved that so many would wish to help him. He then asked me to hug him, so he would recognise it was me, but then I told him it was now time for me to go, until tomorrow, the final healing day.

Day7. Today is the final day of healing, so it was a short session, commencing at 6.53am. I could hear the angels singing above as I surrounded my friend with the golden healing light, as he slept peacefully, so I commenced working on his knees. I removed the blue wraps but I did not open up the wounds. A special blue gel gun, with a curing system attached this time, was handed to me. I inserted the gel each side of the knees, filling any gaps. I was unsure how much to insert but I was told to look at the small screen above the bed, and follow the images. (I had not noticed this screen at any of the other sessions). Each individual leg, once the gel was inserted and cured, had to be straightened and bent at the knee, several times, in order to maintain flexibility, then each knee was wrapped up again for additional support. This bandage will disintegrate in due course, but my friend will not be aware of this happening.

As I stepped back to join the group, I was encouraged to talk to my friend again. As he stirred from his sleep, I told him the sessions are now complete. He thanked me for helping him but I said it was not possible without the help of the whole group of Masters and healers. My pal then commented that they would have not been there if it had not been for me requesting their help. I gave him a hug and told him I needed to go now, but I would send an e-mail.

When we next met, about six months later, I found out that in the middle of the healing sessions, my friend felt so well and free from pain, he actually hauled a huge, heavy gas cylinder onto his property. It was only later that day, did he read my mail telling him, 'light duties only for the time being'. This explained the swelling part way through the treatment. My pal also commented his shoulder too, was also cured and that he no longer relies on pain-killers. I explained that after the psychic procedure, the whole body was healed with the golden light, hence the shoulder improvement too. I told him I always make notes of such happenings and maybe one day, I will let him read them.